Cancer 101

A Witty Guide to Understanding the Big "C"

Ernestine Muanya

DEDICATION

This book is dedicated to two kinds of people. First of all, to all the fighters, survivors and relentless optimists, who have faced the relentless storm of cancer with unwavering courage. To all the curious Johns and Janes out there who just want to know a thing or two about cancer and to navigate its complex labyrinth. This book is dedicated to the quest of knowledge, awareness of what is fact and fiction, and empowerment in the world of a cancer epidemic.
Know better and make positive changes in your lives.

TABLE OT CONTENTS

FIRST THINGS FIRST

Cells are the basic units that make up the human body. The human body is composed of trillions of cells. These cells provide structure for the body, they help take in nutrients from food, they convert those nutrients into energy, and they carry out specialized functions. Cells also contain the body's hereditary material and they can make copies of themselves.

In our lives, as we go about our day, all the cells in our bodies are hard at work. They grow and divide to make new cells as the body needs them. Normally, cells are eventually supposed to die when they get too old or damaged; then, new cells take their place.

Cancer begins when genetic changes happen, and the cell is somehow altered so that it multiplies out of control. Many cancers cause rapid growth of the cells, while others cause cells to grow and divide at a slower rate. Many forms of cancer contribute to noticeable outgrowths called tumors, while others, including leukemia, don't. A tumor is a mass composed of a cluster of such abnormal cells.

Cancer: The Definition in layman terms:
In very simple terms, Cancer is an abnormal condition in the body where the body's cells start to grow uncontrollably. These abnormal cells can go on to form masses or lumps, which are called tumors; and eventually could infiltrate and destroy normal body tissue.

Cancer is the second-leading cause of death in the world. But survival rates are improving for many types of cancer, thanks to improvements in cancer screening, treatment and prevention.

What Causes a Cell to Become Cancerous?
Cancer occurs when genetic mutations or changes to the DNA in abnormal cells, cause them to divide rapidly and abnormally. One can either inherit these mutations or develop them due to environmental factors.

As mutations occur, a cell may gain the ability to grow without restraint and invade nearby tissue— to become, in effect, a cancer cell.

CANCER: HOW IT ALL STARTS

Cancer Risk factors

Certain risk factors may increase your chance of developing cancer. They can include:

- tobacco use
- high alcohol consumption
- an unhealthy diet, characterized by red and processed meat, sugary drinks and salty snacks, starchy foods, and refined carbohydrates including sugars and processed grains.
- a lack of physical activity
- exposure to air pollution
- exposure to radiation
- unprotected exposure to UV light, such as sunlight
- infection by certain viruses including _H. pylori_, human papillomavirus (HPV), hepatitis B, hepatitis C, HIV, and the Epstein-Barr virus, which causes infectious mononucleosis

Of note, as of today, more than 400 chemical agents have been classified as 'carcinogenic', 'probably carcinogenic, or 'possibly carcinogenic' by the IARC (International Agency for Research on Cancer (IARC), a branch of the World Health Organization that monitors cancer occurrence worldwide and performs epidemiological and laboratory investigations to understand the causes of cancer. You can visit their website at: https://www.iarc.who.int/

Carcinogens. What are they?

These are substances, agent, or factors that can cause cancer. Most Carcinogens, by themselves, or in combination, can directly damage the genetic information in our cells, in the DNA, and can cause changes called mutations; leading to a disruption in the normal process of growth and cell division.

In the United States, there are two main organization, who have the power to decide which environmental exposures cause cancer in humans. The National Toxicology Program (NTP), an interagency program of the U.S. Department of Health and Human Services (HHS), and the International Agency for Research on Cancer (IARC), the cancer agency of the World Health Organization. Both the IARC and NTP are said to act independently. It is the NTP that releases the publication; 'Report on Carcinogens' every few years, in which it identifies agents, substances, mixtures, or exposures (collectively called "substances") in the environment that may cause cancer in humans.

Types of carcinogens
Researchers divide carcinogens into three main categories. These include:

- **Chemical carcinogens:** These are carcinogens that people release into the environment through pollution, such as through car exhaust fumes, industrial by-products, and cigarette smoke tobacco). Others are: Radon, Benzene, Formaldehyde, acetaldehyde, asbestos, Ethanol in alcoholic beverages, Ethylene oxide, Etoposide
- **Physical or environmental carcinogens:** These carcinogens come from the environment. UV rays from sunlight and radiation from X-rays or other radioactive materials are examples of physical carcinogens.
- **Oncogenic/Biologic viruses:** These are bacteria, parasites, or viruses that can cause cancer. Examples include human papillomavirus (HPV), Epstein-Barr, and hepatitis B. The fungus Aspergillus flavus growing on stored grains, nuts and peanut butter

It is important to note that:

Carcinogens do not necessarily cause cancer every time someone interacts with them. However, exposure to a carcinogen can raise a person's risk of developing certain cancers.

Just because a substance has been designated as a carcinogen, it does not mean that the substance will necessarily cause cancer.

Many factors influence whether a person exposed to a carcinogen will develop cancer, including the amount and duration of the exposure and the individual's genetic background.

While it is impossible to try to eliminate carcinogen exposure, it is important to try to take steps to reduce what you come in contact with.

TUMORS

A tumor is an abnormal mass of tissue that forms when cells either grow too uncontrollably, or do not die when they should- like in the normal cell cycle. As such, this mass of tissue, has no beneficial function in the body. It is important to take note that, while most cancers will develop to form tumors, not all those tumors will be cancerous.

Benign Versus Malignant

Benign, or noncancerous, tumors do not spread to other parts of the body, and do not create new tumors. Malignant, or cancerous, tumors crowd out healthy cells, interfere with body functions, and draw nutrients from body tissues.

Getting Deeper in the Subject Matter: From symptoms, to biopsy, to diagnosis of Cancer

The journey from symptoms to the work-up process, to diagnose, to treatment is not often straight forward/linear like we would expect it to be. That is because for most cancers, there are no early warning symptoms or signs, and even when the symptoms do appear, there are usually vague, non-specific. So much time is spent on speculation and trying to self-manage these vague symptoms.

A good example is, for example, someone with abdominal symptoms – abdominal bloating, vague abdominal pain, a little anorexia, some indigestion, fatigue- might simply shrug off these symptoms, attributing it to work stress, traumatic period in one's life, a period of unhealthy eating, lack of exercising. It can be difficult for these patients to carefully filter through these symptoms and decipher those that might be related to a cancer from those that are not.

SIGNS / SYMPTOMS OF CANCER

The Signs and symptoms caused by cancer will vary, very widely, depending on the part of the body that is affected. For many, there are no symptoms at all until the cancer has metastasized (spread) to other parts of the body.

Irrespective of the part of the body involved, or the type of cancer; here ate sone wide-ranging signs and symptoms associated with cancer:

- Fatigue
- Weight changes, including unintended loss or gain
- Changes in bowel or bladder habits, blood in the stool
- Difficulty swallowing / Hoarseness/ Cough that does not go away
- Unexplained bleeding or bruising
- Persistent pain. Unexplained muscle or joint pain

Breast Changes:
- Lump or firm feeling in your breast or under your arm
- Nipple changes or discharge
- Skin that is itchy, red, scaly, dimpled, or puckered
- Lump or area of thickening that can be felt under the skin

Skin changes
- A flesh-colored lump that bleeds or turns scaly,
- A new mole or a change in an existing mole
- A sore that does not heal
- Jaundice (yellowing of the skin and whites of the eyes)
- Persistent cough or trouble breathing
- Persistent indigestion or discomfort after eating
- Persistent, unexplained fevers or night sweats

Neurological problems
- Headaches
- Seizures
- Vision changes
- Hearing changes
- Drooping of the face

The Key take-away Points:
If you have symptoms that do not get better after a few weeks, it is important to seek medical counsel so that you can be worked up and if there ae any issues found, they are diagnosed and treated as early as possible.

Unlike popular believe, cancer does not usually cause pain, so do not wait for symptoms of pain as a catalyst to seek medical help.

DIAGNOSING CANCER

How Tissue is Obtained

For a formal diagnosis of cancer to be made, a tissue needs to be obtained through biopsy and a pathologist examines cells or tissues by cutting them into very thin slices, called sections, and examining them closely under a microscope. The specimen must be processed to make it solid before it can be cut into sections. A <u>biopsy specimen</u> can be obtained in several ways, such as by

- taking a tissue sample from the surface of the skin
- using a needle inserted through the skin to withdraw tissue or fluid
- inserting a thin, lighted tube called an <u>endoscope</u> through the mouth, <u>anus</u>, <u>urethra</u>, or a small incision in the skin to look at areas inside the body and remove a sample using special tools that pass through the tube

If the entire mass or cancerous tissue is removed during surgery, the surgeon will typically attempt to remove some normal tissue around the tumor as well(known as the <u>margin</u>) for examination by the pathologist to make sure that it doesn't contain tumor cells.

Special considerations:

*For some cancer types; especially breast cancer and melanoma, the surgeon may also remove nearby lymph nodes, called the <u>sentinel lymph nodes</u> (this is the <u>first lymph node or group of nodes draining a cancer</u>), so the pathologist can see if these contain cancer cells. The presence of absence of cancer cell in these nodes will affect treatment choices.

*Certain molecular tests, sometimes called biomarker tests, are done as part of the initial pathology analysis for all cases of a given cancer type. For example, a pathology report for a patient with suspected breast cancer will include the results of testing for <u>estrogen</u> and <u>progesterone receptors</u> and the protein <u>HER2/neu</u>. Since the different types of breast cancer are treated differently, the results of these tests can help identify what treatments are best for an individual patient.

Tissue and Blood Biopsy

Recently, it has been discovered that tumors shed molecules and cells into bodily fluids and blood and researchers have figured that, studying these molecules and cells can reveal some of the same vital information that tissue biopsies provide. Tissue biopsies require solid matter from the body, usually either directly from a tumor or from bone marrow. A liquid biopsy on the other hand, requires a blood sample taken from the patient. In both types of biopsies, the sample (tissue or blood) is tested for cancer by analyzing genetic material, including tumor cells, cancer cell DNA, almost like a 'fingerprint' of the cancer cell. This helps in tracking the presence of specific mutations associated with cancer to see if patient might can be a candidate for certain targeted treatments or be eligible for certain clinical trials, or to simply better understand their prognosis,

- **Circulating tumor cells (CTCs)**: A CTC is a cancer cell from the tumor that's traveling in your bloodstream.
- **Circulating tumor DNA (catena)**: ctDNA is a DNA fragment from the tumor cell circulating in your blood. DNA contains the genetic code, or instructions, that control a cell's behavior.

Advantages of Liquid Biopsy over Tissue Biopsy

- ✓ Liquid biopsy is considerably less invasive when compared to the tissue biopsy procedure. Liquid biopsies require needle stick to obtain blood, while tissue biopsy may involve a large needle, an <u>endoscope,</u> or open surgery—can be invasive, risky, costly, and painful
- ✓ Test results are typically available much earlier than a standard tissue biopsy, so with liquid biopsy, it is possible to make an early diagnosis.
- ✓ The ease and frequency of the liquid biopsy test offer an advantage over the tissue biopsy. The test can be easily repeated if needed and can be used as often as necessary to monitor the patient's progress.
- ✓ Liquid biopsy is usually much less costly to perform than a tissue biopsy.

- ✓ Some patients may not be able to have a tissue biopsy due to the inaccessibility of their tumors (hard to reach location) or because they have other health conditions that prevent them from undergoing the procedure.
- ✓ Best used for screening, identifying mutations in metastatic cancer, and tracking changes in mutations for treatment

Limitations of Liquid Biopsy Assays:

- ✓ Even though innovative and promising, Liquid biopsy is not yet considered a standard testing procedure as tissue biopsy remains the gold standard for the confirmation and diagnosis of diseases, including various cancers, and for the determination of the characteristics of a disease. Tissue biopsy are still considered the 'traditional/gold standard" method when diagnosing cancer. Best when a known tumor's location is confirmed and available for extraction.
- ✓ There is currently not a widespread utilization of the liquid biopsy test within the medical community. More validation in clinical trials is required on the value of liquid biopsies in the medical setting to support the clinical utility of the test.
- ✓ It is still not clear if the liquid biopsy provides a representative sampling of all genetic clones within a tumor or if there is a bias to specific sub-regions of the tumor.
- ✓ Test sensitivity challenges still exist. Given that circulating tumor cells or DNA are relatively rare compared to the number of hematological molecules found in a blood sample, there are challenges to the test's detection ability (for example, the sensitivity of the liquid biopsy test).

Diagnostic Imaging in Cancer

Diagnostic imaging is basically using medical techniques (X-rays, CT scans, MRIs, Fluoroscopy, ultrasound) to create visual representations of the inside of the body, to help the doctors and other health professional to evaluate, monitor, and even diagnose health conditions. These images are instrumental in providing valued information about the structure, function, and even state, of tissues, organs, bones; thus, helping in identifying any problems or abnormalities.

Not all diagnostic imaging techniques are equal. Some are best at seeing some things more than others.

Uses of Diagnostic Imaging tests In Cancer

- They are sometimes used to look for cancer in its early stages (when it's small and has not spread), and a person has no symptoms. This may be called early detection or cancer screening tests.
- They can be used to look for a mass or lump (tumor) if a person has symptoms. They can also help find out if the symptoms are caused by cancer or by some other type of disease.
- They can sometimes help predict whether a tumor is likely to be cancer. This can help health care providers decide if a biopsy is needed. (In a biopsy, a small piece of tissue is taken out and looked at under the microscope.) A biopsy is almost always needed to know for sure that a change is cancer.
- They can show where the tumor is, even deep inside the body. This helps if a biopsy is needed.
- They can help find out the stage of the cancer (figure out if and/or how far the cancer has spread).
- They can be used to plan treatment, such as showing where radiation therapy beams need to be focused.
- They can show if a tumor has shrunk, stayed the same, or grown after treatment. This can give the cancer care team an idea of how well treatment is working.
- They can help find out if a cancer has come back (recurred) after treatment.

Depending on what you are looking for, Diagnostic Imaging modalities are not all the same.

X-Ray (XR)

Discovered by a German physicist, Wilhelm Roentgen in 1895, this new form of mysterious radiation had the ability to pass through many materials that absorb visible light. He called it 'X'-radiation because he didn't know what it was. X-rays work by sending radiation through the body; areas with high levels of calcium (bones and teeth) blocking the radiation, causing them to appear white on the image; while soft tissues allow the radiation to pass through, causing them to appear gray or black on the image.

- ✓ Ease of use. X-rays easier to use than MRIs or CT scans. There are many portable forms, which makes it an obvious first line option in Emergency rooms and urgent situations, where time is life.
- ✓ Quick to complete. An X-ray is the fastest and most accessible form of imaging; only taking a few minutes to complete.
- ✓ X-rays are ideal for diagnosing issues with bones or the musculoskeletal system: Fractures, Dislocations, Misalignments, Narrowed joint space.

Computed Tomography (CT) Scan

- ✓ Best for diagnosing/examining Blood clots, Stroke, blood system disease, infectious or inflammatory process (ulcerative colitis, Sinusitis), internal bleeding, Bone fractures, including subtle fractures not visible on X-ray, Organ (soft tissue injuries), Kidney/bladder stone.
- ✓ Can create an image of almost the entire body, from the neck to the thighs, in a few seconds, incredibly useful for diagnosing and staging cancer
- ✓ Recommended for patients who are very claustrophobic or cannot have an MRI due to presence of metal implants, pacemakers, implanted devices, some tattoos
- ✓ CT scans are quicker, more widely available and less expensive than MRIs

MRI (Magnetic resonance imaging)

This medical imaging technique uses magnetic field and computer-generated radio waves to create detailed images of the organs and tissues in question. MRIs expose subtle differences between types of tissue and can provide better soft tissue detail than CT scans can.

- ✓ Best suited to examine: Abdomen, Brain, Muscles, Heart, ligaments, tendons, Pelvis, Spine bones, Spinal cord or nerves
- ✓ Spinal cord injury, metastases disease to spine, spinal cord and leptomeningeal disease are best seen on MRI,
- ✓ May be hard to tolerated due to claustrophobia and longer

times in the machine.

✓ Patient with some medical implants, dental implants, some pacemakers, brain stimulator, or other devices/body tattoos may not be cleared for MRI use, as the metallic objects can distort the MRI image and make it difficult to read, due to the powerful magnet inside the machine. Patient's should be educated about this and instructed to notify the team of any devices in their bodies; as well as bring with them any special information card that may have on the device.

The Drawbacks of Diagnostic Imaging

Though tremendously invaluable, Imaging test also have their limits.

✓ By themselves, they cannot always tell for sure if a change is caused by cancer.

✓ Most imaging is only able to detect large groups of cancer cells. No imaging test can show a single cancer cell or even a few. In fact, it takes millions of cells to make a tumor big enough to show up on an imaging test. Meaning that there may be microscopic cells of the cancer roaming about in the blood steam seeking domicile in other parts of the body that we may not be aware of at that time. We have seen in many occasions, were imaging shows new metastatic sites, when just 2 weeks prior, there was nothing noted, and the patient was told everting is fine. Like we say in the oncology, sometimes you cannot see the cancer until it chooses to declare or show itself.

✓ There can be false positives. imaging may identify suspicious areas that, with some work-up and evaluation (biopsy), turn out to be benign. This of course, may cause unnecessary anxiety for anyone.

✓ There is always the concern for radiation exposure. Even though today's imaging devices are safer in terms of the amount of radiation a patient is exposed to, there is still a nagging concern regarding the exposure to any amount of radiation and its potential risk of cancer. This concern is even more magnified for those patients with must go through several of these imaging modalities, for staging, restaging, surveillance, during their lifetime of dealing with the cancer.

Ionizing radiation can damage DNA, and although our cells are equipped to repair most of the damage, they sometimes do the job imperfectly, leaving small areas of "mis-repair." This could result in DNA mutations that may eventually contribute to cancer, down the road.

✓ Adverse Reactions or Side effects to contrast agents could also be an issue. These are Iodine-based and barium-sulfate compounds used in x-ray and CTs, and gadolinium used MRIs exams. These radiocontrast agents or contrast dyes are taken Orally or by IV and help to highlight structures that are difficult to differentiate from their surroundings, such as the brain, spine, liver, or kidneys. Most are iodine-based and are injected intravenously (into a vein) in advance of the scan. Some patients have allergic reaction to them (especially iodine) and may have to be premedicated (prednisone, Benadryl) about 12 to 13 hours before the administration of the contrast for the imaging test.

✓ Can affect the kidney. Kidney or renal dysfunction is a well-known possibility with contrast. Excess iodine is normally removed from the body by the kidneys. However, in patients with unhealthy or impaired kidneys, IV iodinated contrast may worsen kidney function and should be avoided if possible. Other imaging types may be used such as non-contrasted CT, XRs, MRIs.

CANCER STAGING

The 'Stage' of the Cancer' refers to the extent of the cancer; such as how large the tumor is, and if it has spread to other parts of the body. Staging is typically performed at diagnosis after a series of tests (X-Rays, blood work, CTs, MRIs, Bone Scan), and it plays an important role in both diagnosing and treating cancer

When is cancer staged?

Staging does not only occur at the beginning of diagnosis, but it takes places at different phases or intervals throughout the treatment/journey. These include clinical, pathological and post-therapy staging.

Clinical staging: clinical staging is an estimate of the extent of the cancer based on results of physical exams, imaging tests (x-rays, CT scans, etc.), endoscopy exams, and any biopsies that are done before treatment starts. For some cancers, blood tests, are also included in the staging. In clinical staging, a cancer's stage is determined before treatment is started. This helps the oncology team with treatment planning and prognosis.

Pathological staging: Pathologic staging is the standard way to stage certain cancers, especially breast cancer. It is based on a pathologist's study of the tumor tissue and any lymph nodes around the tumor, removed during surgery. Because this information, this staging is considered more accurate.

Post-therapy staging: Post-therapy staging is used in cases where surgery is not the first treatment, but other treatments such as radiation therapy, hormone therapy, chemotherapy, immunotherapy or other therapies are given before surgery. These treatments may be used before surgery to shrink the tumor to make surgery easier. It can help doctors learn how well the cancer/tumor has responded to these treatments, so they will know how to plan ahead. Post-therapy staging is usually indicated with a "y" before the TNM category.

How Cancer is staged

The <u>TNM staging system</u>, is a widely used, globally recognized standard for classifying the extent of spread of cancer, today in the field of oncology, for many solid tumor cancers. There are still other staging systems, which are most specific to a particular type of cancer. Like the TNM, most staging systems must take into consideration these:

- T refers to the size of the original (primary) tumor and whether it has invaded nearby tissue, (Tx, Tis, T0, T1, T2, T3, T4)
- N refers to nearby (regional) lymph nodes that are involved (Nx, N0, N1, N2, N3, N4)
- M refers to whether the cancer has metastasis (spread of cancer from one part of the body to another). M0 means that no distant spread of the cancer has been noted. M1 means that the cancer has been found to have spread to distant tissues or organs.

How many stages of cancer are there?

Most cancers are assigned one of four stages, ranging from stage 1 to 4, with the lowest stage describing early and small tumors and the higher stages categorizing cancers that have progressed and spread to other parts of the body. Stages 1, 2, 3 and 4 may also be written as I, II, III and IV.

- Stage 0 - Indicates a clump of abnormal cells that hasn't spread into neighboring tissue or elsewhere, sometimes called pre-cancer. Surgery often can remove such growths.
- Stage 1, or early-stage or localized cancer: The cancer has not infiltrated deeply into nearby tissue, nor has it spread to lymph nodes or locations away from the primary tumor.
- Stage 2, or early locally advanced cancer: Tumor cells have spread deeper into neighboring tissue, but not to distant sites in the body.
- Stage 3, or advanced-stage or locally advanced cancer: The cancer has grown more deeply into neighboring tissue and spread to lymph nodes but hasn't spread to distant sites in the body.
- Stage 4, or metastatic or advanced cancer: Cancer cells have

spread beyond nearby tissue and into lymph nodes and parts of the body, including organs, potentially far from the original site.

Another staging system divides the cancer into five main categories.

- <u>In situ</u>—Abnormal cells are present but have not spread to nearby tissue.
- <u>Localized</u>—Cancer is limited to the place where it started, with no sign that it has spread.
- <u>Regional</u>—Cancer has spread to nearby lymph nodes, tissues, or organs.
- Distant—Cancer has spread to distant parts of the body.
- Unknown—There is not enough information to figure out the stage.

Note

It is very important to note that each cancer type has its own version of the TNM staging systems; that means the letter and numbers will not mean the same for every type of cancer.

For example, in some cancers, T categories describes the size of the tumor, while in others, it describes how deeply embedded the tumor has grown into the organ it is invading. So, T1 in breast cancer would be different from T1 in lung or colon cancer.

CANCER CLASSIFCATION

Cancers are classified in two ways:
First, by the type of tissue in which the cancer originates (histological type) and secondly, by the primary site, or the location in the body where the cancer first developed.

Histological Classification: Grouped into six major categories:

- <u>Carcinoma</u>: Carcinomas form in epithelial cells; the skin or the tissue that covers the surface of internal organs and glands. They usually form solid tumors and account for 80% to 90% of all cancer diagnoses. They are the most common type of cancer. Examples of carcinomas include <u>prostate cancer</u>, <u>breast cancer</u>, <u>lung cancer</u>, and <u>colorectal cancer</u>.
- <u>Sarcoma</u>
- <u>Myeloma</u>
- <u>Leukemia</u>
- <u>Lymphoma</u>
- <u>Mixed Types</u>

What are the types of carcinoma?

- **<u>Adenocarcinoma</u>** affects organs or glandular tissues, and can cause breast, lung, colorectal, stomach, prostate, pancreatic, and esophageal cancer, among others. Hepatocellular carcinoma (liver cancer), renal cell carcinoma (kidney cancer), cholangiocarcinoma (bile duct cancer) are common types of adenocarcinoma.
- **<u>Basal cell carcinoma</u> (BCC) affects basal cells** (which produce new skin cells), and BCC is the most common type of skin cancer worldwide. It is slow growing and for most people, it is highly treatable, not life-threatening and seldom spreads to other part of the body.
- **<u>Squamous cell carcinoma</u> (SCC)** starts in the epidermis's squamous cell layer (topmost layer of skin cells). It usually

appears in the parts of your skin most exposed to sun (face, ears, neck, arms, legs) as well as in the mucous membranes lining your lungs, esophagus, head and neck. It's the second most common type of skin cancer. SCC generally spreads faster than BSS.

- **<u>Ductal carcinoma in situ (DCIS)</u>** starts in your breast milk ducts. In DCIS, the abnormal cells remain contained (in situ or in place) in the milk ducts (canals that carry milk from the lobules to the nipple openings during breastfeeding), meaning that the carcinoma hasn't spread to cells outside your milk ducts. DCIS is considered noninvasive, pre-invasive, or pre-cancerous.
- **<u>Invasive (infiltrating) ductal carcinoma</u>** starts in your breast milk ducts, like DCIS. Unlike DCIS, invasive ductal carcinoma is 'invasive' and has spread to nearby breast tissue. Invasive ductal carcinoma (IDC), also called infiltrating ductal carcinoma, is the most common type of breast cancer, making up about 75% of all breast cancers.
  - **Sarcomas.** A <u>sarcoma</u> develop from tissue cells called mesenchymal cells that help support and connect the body. A sarcoma can develop in fat, muscles, nerves, tendons, joints, blood vessels, lymph vessels, cartilage, or bone.
  - **Leukemias.** Leukemia is a cancer of the blood and blood marrow. Leukemia begins when healthy blood cells change and grow uncontrollably. The 4 main types of leukemia are <u>acute lymphocytic leukemia,</u> <u>chronic lymphocytic leukemia,</u> <u>acute myeloid leukemia,</u> and <u>chronic myeloid leukemia.</u>
  - **Lymphomas.** Lymphoma is a cancer that begins in the lymphatic system. The lymphatic system is a network of vessels and glands that help fight infection. The 2 main types of lymphomas are <u>Hodgkin lymphoma</u> and <u>non-Hodgkin lymphoma.</u>

METASTASIS

Metastasis is an expression used to describe the spread of cancer beyond where it started. Unlike normal cells, cancer cells can grow outside of the place in the body where they originated.

As carcinoma cells grow and multiply, they form solid masses called tumors. Cancer cells can break away from tumors and spread to other parts of your body (metastasize). Labels for carcinoma describe how much it has spread.
   •   Carcinoma in situ: The carcinoma hasn't spread.
   •   Invasive carcinoma: The carcinoma has spread to surrounding tissue close to where it formed.
   •   Metastatic carcinoma: The carcinoma has spread to other parts of your body.

How cancer Metastasizes or spreads

Metastases is the sequential steps in which some tumor cells first migrate from the primary tumor, penetrate blood vessels, lymph nodes, cell membranes and then colonize distant sites.
   a.   The circulatory system is the primary route of spread to distant organs. Bone and soft tissue tumors (sarcomas) spread primarily through the blood
   b.   The lymphatic vessels also provide a route for travel of the cancer cells. Lymph Nodes; tiny, bean-shaped organs, located in clusters in different parts of the body, such as the neck, groin area, and under the arms. The lymphatic system, a part of the immune system, protects the body from illness-causing invaders, maintains body fluid levels, absorbs digestive tract fats and removes cellular waste. Melanoma, breast, lung and gastrointestinal tumors spread through the lymphatic system.
   c.   Transcoelomic spread is the third route cancer uses to metastasize; This involves the spread of a malignancy into body cavities that occurs via penetrating the surface of the peritoneal, pleural, pericardial, or subarachnoid spaces. Ovarian tumors can spread trans peritoneally to the surface of the liver.

Once these new cancer cells get to the new destination, they get settle or on the new tissue /organ, and then start multiplying/growing there; developing into new tumors. This is known as metastasis. Metastasis is the trademark of cancer that is responsible for the greatest number of cancer-related deaths.

A CLOSER EXAMINATION OF CANCER/TUMORS

Biopsy: A sample of tissue from the tumor is obtained through a biopsy, and the pathologist examines it under a microscope, to decide, first of all, if it is cancer and, secondly, to gather other information about the genetic makeup of the cancer that will help in treatment planning.

Needle biopsies. This general category refers to different biopsies, each using a special needle to collect cells to test an area for cancer.

For instance, in a <u>fine needle aspiration biopsy</u>, the doctor inserts a very thin, hollow needle through the skin to collect a sample of cells and sometimes fluid for examination. This is the simplest type of biopsy. It is often used when a mass can be felt through the skin. A core needle biopsy uses a larger needle to remove a larger tissue sample than a fine needle biopsy. A vacuum-assisted biopsy uses a suction device to collect a tissue sample through a specially designed needle. Your doctor can collect multiple or large samples from the same biopsy site with this method.

Image-guided biopsy. This is the use an imaging technique, such as ultrasound, during a needle biopsy procedure. It is usually performed using a real-time image. In rea time, Image-guided needle biopsy allows the doctor to biopsy suspicious areas that aren't readily seen or felt through the skin (for example, pelvic masses or sensitive regions) The imaging equipment may be:

- <u>Ultrasound</u>
- Fluoroscopy
- <u>Computed tomography (CT) scan</u>
- X-ray
- <u>Magnetic resonance imaging (MRI) scan</u>

Biopsy

Skin biopsy: This is a procedure to remove cells from the surface of your body so that they can be tested in a lab. Skin biopsy procedures include:

a. **Shave biopsy.** Use of razor to scrape the surface of your skin.

b. **Punch biopsy.** Use of a circular tool to remove a small section of the skin's deeper layers.

c. **Incisional biopsy.** Use of a scalpel to remove a small area of skin. Whether you receive stitches to close the biopsy site depends on the amount of skin removed.

d. **Excisional biopsy.** A surgical procedure that removes an entire tumor or area of abnormal skin and some of the surrounding skin. Stitches usually used to close site.

Surgical (excisional) biopsy. This type of biopsy is done under surgery to remove the suspected cancerous tissues.

Laparoscopic biopsy. A diagnostic procedure that uses a small camera and instruments to examine or remove tissues or organs from the abdomen or pelvis. When used for the chest, it is called a thoracoscopy or thoracoscopic biopsy.

Bone marrow aspiration and biopsy. The bone marrow is the spongy-semi-solid tissue found within the spongy portions of bones whose major function is to generate blood cells.

A bone marrow assessment offers detailed information about the condition of the bone marrow and blood cells. Bone marrow aspiration takes a small sample of the liquid portion of the bone marrow, with a needle, while the biopsy takes a sample of solid tissue portion.

Tumor Grade

Tumor grade describes how normal or abnormal cancer cells look under a microscope. The more normal the cells look, the less aggressive the cancer and the more slowly it grows and spreads. On the other hand, the more abnormal the cells look, the more aggressive the cancer and the faster it is likely to grow and spread.

There are 5 classifications of Tumor Grades:

- Grade X: Grade cannot be assessed (undetermined grade)
- Grade 1: Well differentiated (low grade)
- Grade 2: Moderately differentiated (intermediate grade)
- Grade 3: Poorly differentiated (high grade)
- Grade 4: Undifferentiated (high grade)

Take Note:

Tumor grade is not the same thing as cancer stage. Stage refers to how large a cancer tumor is and how far the cancer has spread. See Cancer Staging to learn more.

The knowledge of tumor grades helps the oncology team to formulate a <u>treatment plan</u> and also to estimate prognosis (an estimate or projection of how the disease will respond or the chance of recovery or survival from the disease)

Tumor Markers

These are proteins, mainly found in blood or urine, stool, tumors, which are biochemical indicators of presence of a tumor.

Tumor makers are used as diagnostic tool. There can also be an elevation of some tumor markers in some normal cells, cancerous cells, and in some medical conditions. Also, some slow growing tumors may produce very low amounts of tumor markers. For this reason, oncologist do not rely on tumors markers alone to make oncologic decisions.

Categories of Tumor Markers

There are two (2) main types of tumor markers:

1) Circulating tumor markers (can be found in the blood, urine, stool, or other bodily fluids of some patients with cancer).

   Circulating tumor markers are used to:

   - estimate <u>prognosis</u>
   - determine the <u>stage</u> of cancer
   - detect cancer that remains after treatment (<u>residual disease</u>) or that has returned after treatment
   - assess how well a treatment is working
   - monitor whether the treatment has stopped working

2) Tumor tissue (or cell) markers (found in the actual tumors

themselves).

Tumor tissue markers are used to:

- diagnose, <u>stage</u>, and/or classify cancer
- estimate prognosis
- select an appropriate treatment (e.g., treatment with a <u>targeted therapy</u>)

There is an exhaustive list of tumor markers, but here are some commonly used ones:

Tumor Marker(s)	How it's obtained	How It's used	Cancer Type
CA 15-3, CA 27.29	Blood	To assess whether treatment is working or if the cancer has recurred	Breast Cancer
CEA	Blood	To keep track of how well cancer treatments are working and check if cancer has come back or spread	Colorectal cancer and some other cancers
CA19-9	Blood	To assess whether treatment is working	Pancreatic, gallbladder, bile duct, and gastric cancers
PSA (prostate specific antigen)	Blood	To screen for /diagnose prostate cancer <ul><li>Monitor treatment</li><li>Check to see if cancer has come back after you've finished</li></ul>	prostate cancer

		treatment	
CD20	Blood	To help determine treatment	<u>Non-Hodgkin lymphoma</u>
CgA	Blood	To help in diagnosis, assessment of treatment response, and evaluation of recurrence	<u>Neuroendocrine tumors</u>
Alpha-fetoprotein (AFP)	Blood	Help diagnose liver cancer and follow treatment response.	Liver cancer and <u>germ cell tumors</u>
ALK **gene rearrangements and overexpression**	Tumor		Non-small cell lung cancer, <u>anaplastic large cell lymphoma</u>, <u>histiocytosis</u>
Beta-2-microglobulin (B2M)	Blood, urine, or <u>cerebrospinal fluid</u>	To determine prognosis and follow response to treatment	Multiple myeloma, chronic lymphocytic leukemia, and some lymphomas

MUTATIONS & CANCER

The inherit nature of cancer and tumors to grow and spread. In most cancers, there may be genetic variations that appear to promote the growth of the tumor/cancer. That is why the mutation station of the tumor matters. Mutations happen often. A mutation may be beneficial, harmful, or neutral. This depends where in the gene the change occurs. Typically, the body corrects most mutations.

A single genetic mutation will likely not cause cancer. Usually, cancer occurs from multiple mutations over a lifetime. That is why cancer occurs more often in older people. They have had more opportunities for mutations to build up.

It all starts with the 'Gene'. What are Genes?
Genes, considered the basic unit of inheritance, contained inside each cell as pieces of DNA. Each gene contains the code (instructions) to make a certain protein, and each protein has a specific job. They instruct the cell how to make the proteins it needs to function. For example, some genes code for proteins that help the cell grow and divide to make new cells, while others code for proteins that help keep cell growth under control.

Genetic Mutations: There are 2 Basic Types
1. **Acquired (Somatic) mutations.**
An acquired mutation is 'acquired' during your lifetime. They occur from damage to genes in a cell during a person's life. For example, this could be a breast cell or a colon cell, which then goes on to divide many times and form a tumor. A tumor is an abnormal mass. Age is the biggest risk factor for acquired mutations; the longer we live, the more likely we are to acquire these mutations that happen by chance.

These are the most common cause of cancer. Cancer that occurs because of acquired mutations is called sporadic cancer. Acquired mutations are not found in every cell in the body and they are not passed from parent to child.

Factors that cause these mutations include:

- Tobacco
- Ultraviolet (UV) radiation
- Viruses
- Age

2. **Germline (Hereditary) Mutations**.

The germline mutation is present in the DNA in the egg or sperm at the time of conception and exists in every cell of your body. It passes directly from one or both parents, to a child at the time of conception. As the embryo grows into a baby, the mutation from the initial sperm or egg cell is copied into every cell within the body. Because the mutation affects reproductive cells, it can pass from generation to generation.

Cancer caused by germline mutations is called inherited cancer. These are less common, accounting for about 5% to 20% of all cancers.

For example

PIK3CA gene mutations are common in <u>breast cancer</u>, occurring in roughly 30% to 40% of tumors, and most commonly found in estrogen receptor-positive breast cancer.

Around 5% of people with cancer have a point mutation in the KRAS gene that replaces the DNA letter G with an A. This single letter change creates an abnormal KRAS protein that constantly tells cells to grow, leading to cancer.

Inheriting damaged copies of the BRCA1 or BRCA2 genes can increase the risk for breast cancer and ovarian cancer in women and the risk for breast and prostate cancer in men, as well as many other cancers (Cervical cancer, Uterine cancer, Colon cancer, Pancreatic cancer, Gallbladder cancer or bile duct cancer, Stomach cancer

Melanoma)

<u>Important to know:</u>

Also known as 'Molecular profiling' or 'Cancer genomic sequencing, tumor sequencing is important for cancer patients. It involves a process of scrutinizing the genetic material of a cancerous tumor to recognize specific genetic mutations, variations or alteration. It is a great tool in the oncology as it helps to tailor oncology treatments to individual patients and thereby improving their outcomes. Personalized cancer treatment is thus a move away from the one-size-fits-all treatment approach that is determined by the individual's tumor characteristics which is identified by tumor sequencing, in order to improve efficacy of response, quality of life, and be more targeted to the tumor without causing collateral damage to the normal cells.

In addition, the chemotherapy when scientifically complemented by the right natural supplements selected based on chemo and cancer characteristics (identified by tumor sequencing) can further improve the odds of success and well-being of the cancer patient.

Routine testing for these biomarkers is not currently recommended or standard of care in the start of therapy. However, once diagnosed with stage IV/ metastatic cancer or there is disease progression on initial standard therapy, the oncology team can order a biomarker panel testing done on the tumor itself through Next Generation Sequencing (NGS).

Tumor Suppressor Genes

Cancer is a complex genetic disorder exhibiting considerable variability and so, we cannot find a definite cure for cancer without looking at the role of Tumor Suppressor Genes. Also called Anti-oncogene, Tumor suppressor genes are present in all cells (somatic cells; cells in the body that are not involved in sexual reproduction) in our body. These genes make special proteins that put the brakes on cell growth that may cause cancer and at the molecular level, these genes work by synthesizing proteins that control cell differentiation, growth, reproduction and longevity, thus they play an important role in preventing the development of cancer cells.

When tumor suppressor genes are altered or inactivated due to a mutation (either one that is present at birth or one that occurs later in life), they make proteins that are less effective at controlling cell growth and/or repair; resulting in unrestrained growth of damaged or abnormal cells, which leads to uncontrolled growth and the development of cancerous tumors.

Examples of tumor suppressor genes: Please see table below.

Gene	Original Gene Function	Two-Hit Hypothesis	Carcinomas caused by their mutations
p53	Apoptosis	No	Half of all known malignancies
BRCA 2	Cell division and death, and repair of double-stranded DNA breaks	Yes	Breast/Ovarian/Prostrate cancer. To lesser degree, Male breast cancer, prostrate/Pancreatic/Melanoma
BRCA 1	work to repair damaged DNA.	Yes	Breast /Ovarian cancer
VHL	Cell division, death, and differentiation	Yes	Kidney Cancer
APC	DNA damage, cell division, migration, adhesion, death	Yes	Colorectal Cancer
Rb	DNA Replication, cell division and death	Yes	Retinoblastoma
NF1	Cell differentiation, division,	No	Nerve tumors, Neuroblastoma

	development, RAS signal transduction		
<u>PTCH</u>	provides instructions for producing the patched-1 protein, which functions as a receptor.	No	Medulloblastoma, Basal Cell Carcinoma
PTE N	Works in the regulation of the <u>cell cycle</u>, preventing cells from growing and dividing too rapidly. mutation in the *PTEN* gene is caused by a condition called Cowden syndrome.		glioblastoma, lung cancer, breast cancer, and prostate cancer, Uterine cancer, kidney cancer, Thyroid cancer, Colorectal (colon and rectal) cancer and colon polyps

*Two-hit hypothesis: Initially proposed by Alfred Knudson in 1971. It suggests that for some genetic mutations, two distinct genetic 'hits' are required to cause the disease. the Theorize that both alleles that code for a particular protein must be affected before an effect is manifested

Take Particular Note:
The most mutated gene in people with cancer is *p53* or *TP53 are*

*the most mutated gene in people with cancer, with m*ore than 50% of cancers involve a missing or damaged *p53* gene.

-Most *p53* gene mutations are acquired. Germline *p53* mutations are rare, but patients who carry them are at a higher risk of developing many different types of cancer.

-Mutations to the BRCA1 and BRCA2 genes are inherited, either from a person's mother or father (or both), and these are linked to an increased risk for several types of cancer—most notably, female breast and ovarian cancers.

Proto-oncogenes

Proto-oncogenes are genes that normally help cells grow and divide to make new cells, or to help cells stay alive in a well-controlled cycle. They do this by encoding proteins involved in signal transduction and cell cycle.

Proto-oncogenes Examples

- Ras: The first proto-oncogene to be shown to turn into an oncogene is called Ras.
- HER2: Stands for Human Epidermal Growth Factor Receptor 2; a protein found on the surface of some cancer cells. It is another well-known proto-oncogene is HER2.
- Myc: The Myc gene is associated with a type of cancer called Burkitt's lymphoma.
- Cyclin D. Cyclin D is another proto-oncogene.

From Proto-oncogenes to Oncogenes

When a proto-oncogene mutates (changes) or there are too many copies of it (amplification) due to DNA damage, it can become turned on (activated) when it is not supposed to be, at which point it's now called an oncogene. When this happens, the cell can start to grow out of control, which might lead to cancer. Simply put, proto-oncogenes become oncogenes (which are cancer-producing genes), due to mutations or increased expression that lead to uncontrolled cell division, inhibit cell differentiation, and halt cell death. Oncogenes are mutated genes that can contribute to the development of cancer.

Apart from mutations which are listed earlier and known to cause cancers, there are also some viruses which are considered oncogenic; meaning they can cause or give rise to tumors

Oncogenic DNA viruses include EBV, hepatitis B virus (HBV), human papillomavirus (HPV), human herpesvirus-8 (HHV-8), and Merkel cell polyomavirus (MCPyV). Oncogenic RNA viruses include, hepatitis C virus (HCV) and human T-cell lymphotropic virus-1 (HTLV-1).

Oncogene	Oncogene Function	Cancers Caused by these Oncogenes
RAS	*Ras* is one of the on-and-off switches in a pathway that leads to cell growth. When *Ras* mutates, it encodes for a protein that causes an uncontrolled growth-promoting signal	causes about 30 percent of cancers. Some including colon /pancreatic / lung carcinoma and lung tumors, thyroid tumors
BRAF	BRAF is a gene found on chromosome seven that encodes a protein also called BRAF. The BRAF gene makes a protein that helps control cell growth. It's known as an oncogene. An oncogene works like a gas pedal on a car. Normally, an oncogene turns on cell growth as needed.	Melanoma (1/2 of all melanomas have the BRAF gene mutation) Hairy cell leukemia, Non-Hodgkin lymphoma, Thyroid cancer Ovarian cancer, Lung adenocarcinoma Colorectal cancer Certain brain cancers, including glioblastoma, pilocytic astrocytoma, and pediatric low-grade glioma
HER2	The HER2 gene makes the HER2 protein, a protein with helps control healthy breast cell division and growth. Extra copies	breast cancer and ovarian cancer cells.

	of this gene may lead to an excess of HER2 protein, which causes cells to grow more quickly.	
Cyclin D	Works to deactivate a protein called the Rb tumor suppressor. When Cyclin D mutates, it can no longer accomplish this, causing uncontrollable cell growth.	pancreatic cancer, lung cancer, breast cancer, melanoma
Myc	This occurs as the result of chromosomal translocation (unusual rearrangement of chromosomes); a chromosome breaks and part of it reattaches to another chromosome. In Burkitt's lymphoma, a section of a gene that enhances gene function gets moved near the Myc proto-oncogene.	Associated with Burkitt's lymphoma (a severe form of non-Hodgkin's lymphoma).

Reducing Cancer Risk with BRCA1 or BRCA2 gene mutation

There are several options available for reducing cancer risk in individuals who have inherited a harmful BRCA1 or BRCA2 variant.

Increased Screening:

1) Learn to be aware of changes in your breasts beginning at age

18.

2) Breast exam by doctor every 6-12 months beginning at age 25.

3) Yearly breast MRI with contrast (or mammogram if MRI is unavailable) beginning at age 25 and continuing until age 75.

4) Yearly mammogram (for those with average/general risk) beginning at age 40 until age 75.

5) Screening after age 75 should be considered on an individual basis.

6) For Ovarian Cancer: use of transvaginal ultrasound and a CA-125 blood test has not shown benefit and is not recommended.

7) For Pancreatic cancer: All patients with a BRCA mutation regardless of family history of pancreatic cancer, should undergo annual screening for pancreatic cancer with MRI/MRCP or EUS beginning at age 50 (or 10 years earlier than the earliest pancreatic cancer in the family).

8) For Prostate cancer: Begin prostate cancer screening at age 40 with an annual digital rectal exam and Prostate Specific Antigen (PSA) test.

9) For Melanoma: NCCN does not include guidelines for melanoma screening for people with BRCA2 mutations. However, some experts recommend general melanoma risk management such as a yearly full-body skin exam, a yearly eye exam and avoiding too much sun exposure.

Many patients have questions the potential harmful effects of these screening modalities. For example, some people argue that the MRI is notorious for resulting in false-positive results for breast masses and that the women who already have a harmful BRCA variant might be particularly sensitive to the DNA-damaging effects of tests that involve radiation (such as mammography) because they already have a defect in DNA repair. All of these are legit concerns, however, the benefits of catching the cancer on time, and knowing what to do, far outweighs the negatives.

Risk-Reduction Surgery. Risk-reducing, or prophylactic, surgery involves removing as much of the "at-risk" tissue as possible. Women may choose to have both breasts removed (bilateral risk-reducing mastectomy) to reduce their risk of breast cancer. Surgery to remove a woman's ovaries and fallopian tubes (bilateral risk-reducing salpingo-oophorectomy) can help reduce her risk of ovarian cancer. (Ovarian cancers often originate in the fallopian tubes, so it is essential that they be removed along with the ovaries.) Removing the ovaries may also reduce the risk of breast cancer in premenopausal women by eliminating a source of hormones that can fuel the growth of some types of breast cancer.

It is important to note that:

> These surgeries are irreversible, and each has potential complications or harms. These include bleeding or infection, anxiety and concerns about body image (bilateral risk-reducing mastectomy), and early menopause in premenopausal women (bilateral risk-reducing salpingo-oophorectomy).

> These Risk-reducing surgery does not guarantee that cancer will not develop because not all at-risk tissue can be removed by these procedures. That is why these surgical procedures are described as "risk-reducing" rather than "preventive." Some women have developed breast cancer, ovarian cancer, or primary peritoneal carcinomatosis (a type of cancer similar to ovarian cancer) even after risk-reducing surgery. Nevertheless, these surgical procedures greatly reduce risk.

> The reduction in breast and ovarian cancer risk from removal of the ovaries and fallopian tubes appears to be similar for carriers of both the BRCA1 and BRCA2 variants.

Chemoprevention. Chemoprevention is the use of medicines to reduce the risk of cancer. Two chemo preventive drugs (tamoxifen [Nolvadex] and raloxifene [Evista]) have been approved by the Food and Drug Administration (FDA) to reduce the risk of breast cancer in women at increased risk.

The potential harms of these drugs include menopausal symptoms, blood clots, stroke, increased risk of endometrial cancer (tamoxifen), and allergic reactions (raloxifene).

CANCER TREATMENTS

During the past decades, we have witnessed many milestone discoveries and advancements in our efforts to make progress against cancer. With targeted therapies, new technological approaches in medicine, and improvements in conventional treatments like chemotherapy, research is moving forward in ways that are bringing hope to families and ensuring a better quality of life for more patients diagnosed with cancer

Personalization of Cancer Treatment

For years, cancer treatment was a cookie-cutter process. Today, treating cancer is all about 'Personalized medicine'. Also known as Precision Medicine' or 'Pharmacogenetics', it is a new innovative way to fight cancer in which treatment is driven by characterization of tumor, genetic characteristics of the patient, microenvironment and host characteristics patient's genes and what is driving their specific disease.

There are many types of cancer treatments. The type of treatment, the cycles, and the order of the treatments, will depend on a whole host of factors: the type of cancer, how advanced the cancer is, and the functional status of the patient. Some people with cancer will have only one or two treatment, while most will receive a combination of treatments.

Cancer treatment options include Surgery, Chemotherapy, Radiation therapy, Immunotherapy, Targeted Therapy, Hormone Therapy, and Stem cell transplants. There are also Clinical trials might also be an option for those who qualify.

I.   Chemotherapy:

Chemotherapy is a systemic medication (travels through the blood stream and reaches all parts of the body) that uses anti-cancer drugs to destroy cancer cells, thereby, keeping cancer cells from growing, dividing, and making more cells. Chemotherapy is 'Cytotoxic', meaning 'toxic to cells' and since it is 'systemic', meaning carried everywhere, it not only affects the cancer cells, but also affect some of the healthy cells in the body. The healthy cells usually recover from the damage (at least most of them), but Cancer cells cannot recover, and so, they eventually die.

Common side effects of chemotherapy drugs include:

Nausea	Vomiting
Diarrhea	Hair loss
Hair loss	Loss of appetite
Fatigue	Fever
Mouth sores	Pain
Constipation	Numbness and Tingling in the fingers/toes

Many of these side effects can be prevented or managed; and most side effects do subside after treatment ends.

Long-lasting and late-developing side effects

Chemotherapy drugs can also cause side effects that don't become evident until months or even years after treatment. Late side effects vary depending on the chemotherapy drug but can include:

Damage to lung tissue
Heart problems
Fertility problems
Kidney problems
Nerve damage (peripheral neuropathy)
Risk of a second cancer

II.   Targeted Therapy

Cancer researchers have discovered some of the differences within cancer cells that enable them to thrive. Targeted therapy also called 'precision medicine' or 'personalized medicine', is cancer drugs that work by targeting the differences in cancer cells that help them to grow and survive. They provide a 'targeted' approach, aimed at inhibiting molecular pathways that are critical to tumor growth and maintenance, altering the inner workings of the cell, focusing on the part of the cancer cell that makes it different from the normal, healthy cell.

a. **Angiogenesis Inhibitors:** They work by blocking the formation of new blood vessels that feed and nourish the cancer cells. Example: bevacizumab (many different cancers).

b. **Monoclonal antibodies☐ :** These might deliver molecules by themselves or molecules with drugs into or onto the cancer cell to kill it. Monoclonal antibodies can be classified as targeted therapy or immunotherapy, depending on the type of monoclonal antibody. For example, HER2-targeted Agents: Trastuzumab (Herceptin), Pertuzumab (Perjeta).

c. **Anti-CD20 Monoclonal Antibodies**: monoclonal antibodies: these drugs target a protein called CD20 found on some B-cell leukemia and non-Hodgkin lymphomas. E.g.: Rituximab, Obinutuzumab

d. **Proteasome Inhibitors**: These disrupt normal cell functions so the cancer cells die. Example: bortezomib (multiple myeloma)

e. Small molecule inhibitors: These drugs are small enough to get inside cancer cells and block certain proteins that tell cancer cells to grow.

Types of small molecule inhibitors include:

- **Signal transduction inhibitors** or TKIs Tyrosine kinase inhibitors (TKIs) block proteins called tyrosine kinases from sending signals that tell cancer cells to grow, multiply and spread. Without this signal, the cancer cells may die.

e.g.: axitinib (Inlyta), dasatinib (Sprycel), erlotinib (Tarceva), imatinib (Glivec), nilotinib (Tasigna), pazopanib (Votrient), sunitinib (Sutent)

- **mTOR inhibitors**: These drugs block mammalian target of rapamycin (mTOR), a protein that tells cancer cells to grow and spread. e.g: Afinitor (Everolimus).
- **PARP inhibitors** These drugs block poly (ADP-ribose) polymerase (PARP), a protein that repairs damaged DNA in cancer cells. e.g.: Olaparib
- **CDK inhibitors** These drugs target and block cyclin-dependent kinase (CDK) from sending signals that tell cancer cells to grow, multiply and spread. Without this signal, the cancer cells will die.

CDK4/6: Ibrance (Palbociclib), Kisqali (Ribociclib), Verzinio (Abemaciclib).

Pan-DCK Inhibitors: these inhibit a wider range of cyclin-dependent kinase compared to CDK4/6. Since they have a more generalized effect on call cycle control, they could be effective to various types of cancer. e.g: Flavopiridol and Dinaciclib.

III.   Immunotherapy

Immunotherapy use the body's own immune system to fight cancer cells by stimulating the immune systemin. They work to stimulate a host response that effectuates long-lived tumor destruction Monoclonal antibodies and immune checkpoint inhibitors

Antibodies are found naturally in our blood and help us to fight infection. MAB therapies mimic natural antibodies but are made in a laboratory. 'Monoclonal' just means they are all one type. Each MAB recognizes one particular protein and they work by first recognizing and finding specific proteins on the cancer cells, and then they proceed bind to cancer cells and block their ability to grow and divide, or even mark them for destruction by the immune system. For example, trastuzumab (Herceptin) is a monoclonal antibody that targets HER2-positive breast cancer cells and can be used in combination with chemotherapy to improve survival rates.

a. Immune Checkpoint Inhibitors

The immune system relies on T cells to fight cancer. These specialized cells are extremely powerful and have the potential to also damage healthy cells. So, normally, when the body's immune system is attacking pathogens, immune checkpoint molecules control T cells activity through immune checkpoints, thereby, protecting the normal tissues from damage.

Checkpoint inhibitors work by releasing a natural brake on your immune system so that immune cells called T cells recognize and continue to attack tumors. This therapy is sometimes called immune checkpoint blockade because the molecule that acts as a brake on immune cells — the checkpoint — is blocked by the drug.

For example, an immune checkpoint protein called CTLA-4 shuts a T cell off to prevent it from accidentally damaging healthy cells. So, in the presence of cancer, by blocking CTLA-4, scientists allowed T cells to continue working and eliminate cancer.

PD-1 Inhibitors
Pembrolizumab (Keytruda)
Nivolumab (Opdivo)
Cemiplimab (Libtayo)

PD-L1 Inhibitors
Atezolizumab (Tecentriq)
Avelumab (Bavencio)
Durvalumab (Imfinzi)

CTLA-4 Inhibitors
Ipilimumab (Yervoy)
Tremelimumab (Imjuno)

LAG-3 Inhibitors
Relatlimab. This drug is given along with the PD-1 inhibitor nivolumab (in a combination known as Opdualag).

b. Oncolytic Virus therapy
Viruses are particles that infect or enter our cells and then use the

cell's own genetic machinery to make copies of themselves and subsequently spread to surrounding uninfected cells. With that knowledge, Oncolytic Virus is a genetically engineered or naturally existing virus that can selectively replicate in cancer cells and then kill them without damaging the healthy cells.

To date, only one oncolytic virus—a genetically modified form of a herpesvirus for treating melanoma—has been approved by the Food and Drug Administration (FDA), though some viruses are being evaluated as potential treatments for cancer in clinical trials.

c. T-cell therapy

T-cell transfer therapy is a type of immunotherapy that makes your own immune cells better able to attack cancer. There are two main types of T-cell transfer therapy: tumor-infiltrating lymphocytes (or TIL) therapy and CAR T-cell therapy. Both involve collecting your own immune cells, growing large numbers of these cells in the lab, and then giving the cells back to you through a needle in your vein. T-cell transfer therapy is also called adoptive cell therapy, adoptive immunotherapy, and immune cell therapy.

d. Cancer Vaccines

Cancer vaccines are just another frontier in the use of immunotherapy to fight cancer which work like all vaccine do, by training your immune system to defend your body against foreign invaders or abnormal cells that pose a threat. There are two main types of cancer vaccines:

➢ **Preventive Cancer Vaccines:**
- Cervarix, Gardasil vaccines for HPV
- Heplisav-B vaccines for Hepatitis B vaccine)

➢ **Therapeutic Cancer Vaccines:**

These can (1) Stop a tumor from growing or spreading, (2) Destroy cancer cells still in the body after initial treatments like surgery or radiation therapy. (3) for maintenance; to Keep cancer from coming back after treatment.

- Prostate Cancer Vaccine

Sipuleucel-T (Provenge®) a vaccine composed of patients' own stimulated dendritic cells; approved for the treatment of people whose prostate cancer has metastasized (spread). Provenge is created by removing some immune cells, exposing them to a molecule from prostate cancer cells, and then infusing them back into the body.

- Bladder Cancer Vaccines

Bacillus Calmette-Guérin (BCG): a vaccine that uses weakened bacteria to stimulate the immune system; approved for patients with early-stage bladder cancer. BCG is put into the bladder as a liquid through a catheter (a thin, flexible tube), it helps stimulate immune system cells, which then attack the bladder cancer cells.

Nadofaragene firadonevec (Adstiladrin®) is approved for treatment of early-stage bladder cancers that have progressed despite BCG therapy. It consists of an engineered, weakened virus that activates an immune response in the bladder. Like BCG, it is delivered into the bladder through a catheter.

- Melanoma Vaccine

T-VEC (Imlygic®) is an oncolytic virus-based vaccine (see below) that is used to treat advanced melanoma that cannot be completely removed with surgery. It is made of a virus that has been genetically modified to promote an anticancer immune response.

Tumor Heterogeneity

Tumor heterogeneity is one of the major problems limiting the efficacy of targeted therapies and compromising treatment outcomes. heterogeneity in cancer is not limited to differences between different patients, but also occurs within a single patient.

1. **Intertumor heterogeneity**, is the differences between the same tumors in different patients. This is the focus of many cancer studies, contributes to differential patient responses to therapy and is the basis for precision medicine approaches.
2. **Intersite heterogeneity**, which describes differences between distinct tumors within an individual patient (e.g., between the same tumor at the primary site, versus at the metastatic sites).
3. **Intratumor heterogeneity**, refers to differences in cellular morphology, gene expression, metabolism, proliferation, motility and even metastatic potential, in the cells of the same tumor.

Why Heterogeneity is a concern in cancer

The molecular profile of cancer can change over time, which we are not able to monitor with existing strategies using tumor tissue biopsies as the gold standard for molecular diagnostics. For example in a typical breast cancer patient; the initial tumor markers in the initial breast tumor could be ER+PR+HER2 and in the midst of good cancer treatments, the disease progresses to the bone and liver; and biopsy of these site might show a triple negative cancer (ER-PR-HER2-). There are also some patients whose disease are simply refractory to any anti-neoplastic treatments you throw at them.

That is why most patients with advanced cancers treated with appropriately selected targeted therapies become resistant to the therapy, ultimately developing disease progression and succumbing to metastatic disease.

Tumor heterogeneity presents resistant to treatment that is not responsive to matching targeted therapy. Thus, targeting only one abnormality might not be sufficiently lethal for most, if not, all cancer cells.

CANCER SCREENING

Cancer screening is the process of looking for cancer before a person has any symptoms. Screening tests can help find cancer at an early stage, before symptoms appear. When cancer or abnormal tissue is found early, it may be easier to treat or cure. On the other end, by the time symptoms appear, the cancer may have grown and spread or metastasize.

Screening Tools

There are tools used to test or detect pre-cancerous or cancerous conditions in individuals who otherwise do not have any symptoms. The goal of screening has always been to detect cancer, if present, at a very early stage, which could make treatable and or curable.

- ✓ High-quality mammography
- ✓ Ultrasound
- ✓ MRI (Magnetic Resonance Imaging)
- ✓ Clinical breast exam
- ✓ Breast self-exam
- ✓ Colonoscopy
- ✓ CT Scans
- ✓ Skin Exams
- ✓ BRCA Gene Testing
- ✓ Blood Tests
- ✓ HPV test
- ✓ Pap Test

The United States Preventive Services Task Force (USPSTF) and the American Cancer Society (ACS) provide recommendations for cancer screening.

Breast Cancer

- ➢ Women with average or general risk factors, have a screening mammogram every year starting at age 40 and continue to do so, as long as they are in good health, and would want the breast cancer to be treated.

> ➤ All women should have a physical exam of the breasts by a doctor every year and do a breast self-exam every month

> ➤ All people who identify as transgender or gender non-conforming should talk to a doctor about a breast cancer screening schedule that makes sense for them

> ➤ Women with a higher-than-average risk of breast cancer should have a physical exam every six to 12 months.

> ➤ Screening should start before age 40 and include an annual mammogram or breast MRI. The guidelines also say that if a family member has been diagnosed with breast cancer, you should start breast cancer screening when you're seven to 10 years younger than your family member was when she or he was diagnosed. For example, if a family member was diagnosed at age 45, you should start screening between the ages of 35 and 38.

Cervical Cancer Testing

> ➤ For Ages 21-29: to get the first Pap test at age 21, followed by Pap testing every 3 years. Even for the sexually active females, they are not required to get a Pap test before age 21.

> ➤ For Ages 30-65: To get the HPV test every 5 years, HPV/Pap every 5 years, and Pap test every 3 years

> ➤ Note: For those 25-65, testing with an HPV/Pap every 5 years or with a Pap test every 3 years is still acceptable.

> ➤ Older than 65 years: Discuss with your health care provider/team to learn if screening is still needed.

> ➤ If you have been screened regularly and had normal test results, you'll most likely be advised that you that you no longer need screening.

> ➤ If your recent test results were <u>abnormal</u> or you have not been screened regularly, you may need to continue screening beyond age 65.

Colon Cancer

<u>Colon cancer</u> is the second-leading cancer killer of men and women combined and is among the most difficult to detect because it lacks symptoms in early stages.

Starting at age 45, routine screening for colorectal cancer is recommended for almost everyone

> Colonoscopy: This is the use of a long flexible tube (colonoscope) that has a light and tiny camera at the tip, to examine the inside of the colon. It is inserted through the rectum and moved into the colon. It examines the entire large intestines up to the end of the small bowel. 1st colonoscopy should be done at the age of 45, if you are at average risk for colorectal cancer. If no polyps or abnormalities are found, then the next one can be in 10 years. On average every 7 to 10 years.

> Annual fecal occult blood tests (FOBT) or fecal immunochemical tests (FIT). It detects hidden blood in the stool and helps detect early signs of cancer in the bowel.

> Flexible Sigmoidoscopy: Used to examine the lower portion of the colon and rectum (rectum and sigmoid colon). Recommended every 5 years or every 10 years with a FIT every year.

> Stool DNA test: Looks for DNA changes and small amounts of blood shed into the stool. It is a non-invasive test for adults 45 and older, with average risk for colon cancer. Every three years

> Virtual colonoscopy: special X-ray examination of the colon using low dose computed tomography. It is less invasive that conventional colonoscopy. Should be done every 5 years

> Double-contrast barium enema: Done by instilling radiopaque barium to coat the mucosal surface of the colon followed by insufflation of air. Done every 5 to 10 years.

Lung Cancer

The U.S. Preventive Services Task Force (USPSTF) recommends yearly lung cancer screening with LDCT for people who:

> Have a 20 pack-year or more smoking history

> Smoke now or have quit within the past 15 years

> Are between the age of 50 and 80 years old.

Screening tool(s): Low-Dose Computed Tomography (LDCT) Scans

Prostate Cancer

One in seven men will develop <u>prostate cancer</u> in his lifetime.
- Age 50 for men who are at average risk of prostate cancer and are expected to live at least 10 more years.
- Age 45 for men at high risk of developing prostate cancer. This includes African Americans and men who have a first-degree relative (father or brother) diagnosed with prostate cancer at an early age (younger than age 65).
- Age 40 for men at even higher risk (those with more than one first-degree relative who had prostate cancer at an early age).

Screening Tool(s): A prostate-specific antigen (PSA) and Digital rectal Exam (DRE)

Skin Cancer

Check your skin once a month for any changes in moles or other marks, which may indicate a developing <u>skin cancer</u>. If you notice any changes to your skin, tell your doctor right away.

Testicular Cancer

Men should self-check their testicles for any pain, discomfort, or abnormal lumps monthly. <u>Testicular cancer</u>, commonly diagnosed in men ages 20 to 39, has been increasing for several decades. If treated early, testicular cancer patients have a 99 percent survival rate after five years.

The Galleri Test

This is another new way that claims to be efficient in detecting cancer. The Galleri test is a multicancer early detection blood test used to identify more than 50 cancer types in asymptomatic adults 50 years or old Instead of searching for any one type of cancer, it screens an individual for multiple cancers. Its potential is to change the current screening process from screening for individual cancers to one where individuals are screened for multiple cancers with a single blood test.

Other Screening Tests

Screening tests that have not been shown to be effective may still be offered, especially to people who are known to be at increased risk of certain cancers.

a) Alpha-fetoprotein blood test: This test is sometimes used, along with ultrasound of the liver, to try to detect liver cancer early in people at high risk of the disease.

b) Breast MRI: A breast MRI imaging test is often used for women who carry a harmful mutation in the BRCA1 gene or the BRCA2 gene; these mutations increase the risk of breast cancer, as well as other cancers.

c) The CA-125 blood test, which is often done together with a transvaginal ultrasound, may be used to try to detect ovarian cancer early, especially in women with an increased risk of the disease. Although this test can help to diagnose ovarian cancer in women who have symptoms and can be used to evaluate the recurrence of cancer in women previously diagnosed with the disease, it has not been shown to be an effective ovarian cancer screening test.

d) Clinical breast exams and regular breast self-exams

- Routine examination of the breasts by health care providers (clinical breast exam) or by women themselves (breast self-exam) has not been shown to reduce deaths from breast cancer. However, if a woman or her health care provider notices a lump or other unusual change in the breast, it is important to get it checked out.

e. Multi-cancer detection (MCD) tests: In the absence of symptoms, cancer cells can produce such as circulating tumor cells, tumor DNA, and other analytes – that may suggest the presence of cancer in the blood or body fluid. MCDs are new innovative tests that can measure or detect these signals.

f. PSA test: The prostate-specific antigen blood test has been used, often along with a digital rectal exam, for prostate cancer screening. However, expert groups no longer recommend routine PSA testing for most men because many prostate cancers detected with PSA testing are not deadly, and early detection and treatment of PSA-detected cancers has not been shown to reduce the chance of dying from prostate cancer.

g. Skin exams: According to the CDC, skin cancer overall, is the most common type of cancer in the US. Doctors often recommend that people who are at risk for skin cancer examine their skin regularly or have a health care provider do so. It is important to know your skin and be acutely aware of changes in your skin, such as a new mole or a change to an existing mole, and report these to their doctor promptly.

h. Transvaginal ultrasound: The transvaginal ultrasound imaging test, which can create pictures of a woman's ovaries and uterus, is sometimes used in women who are at increased risk of ovarian cancer (because they carry a harmful BRCA1 or BRCA2 gene mutation) or of endometrial cancer (because they have a condition called Lynch syndrome). But it has not been shown to reduce deaths from either cancer.

CANCER PREVENTION: KNOWLEDGE IS POWER

Doctors have identified several ways to reduce your risk of cancer, such as:

- Stop smoking. If you smoke, quit. If you don't smoke, don't start. Smoking is linked to several types of cancer — not just lung cancer. Stopping now will reduce your risk of cancer in the future.
- Avoid excessive sun exposure. Harmful ultraviolet (UV) rays from the sun can increase your risk of skin cancer. Limit your sun exposure by staying in the shade, wearing protective clothing or applying sunscreen.
- Eat a healthy diet. Choose a diet rich in fruits and vegetables. Select whole grains and lean proteins. Limit your intake of processed meats.
- Exercise most days of the week. Regular exercise is linked to a lower risk of cancer. Aim for at least 30 minutes of exercise most days of the week. If you haven't been exercising regularly, start out slowly and work your way up to 30 minutes or longer.
- Maintain a healthy weight. Being overweight or obese may increase your risk of cancer. Work to achieve and maintain a healthy weight through a combination of a healthy diet and regular exercise.
- Drink alcohol in moderation, if you choose to drink. If you choose to drink alcohol, do so in moderation. For healthy adults, that means up to one drink a day for women and up to two drinks a day for men.
- Schedule cancer screening exams. Talk to your doctor about what types of cancer screening exams are best for you based on your risk factors.
- Ask your doctor about immunizations. Certain viruses

increase your risk of cancer. Immunizations may help prevent those viruses, including hepatitis B, which increases the risk of liver cancer, and human papillomavirus (HPV), which increases the risk of cervical cancer and other cancers. Ask your doctor whether immunization against these viruses is appropriate for you.

COMMONE CANCER TERMINOLOGY

Common Cancer Terminology
1) **Active surveillance**: Watching a patient's condition closely without giving them any treatment. During active surveillance, certain exams and tests are done regularly. If there are changes to these test results, treatment may be recommended. Active surveillance may be part of a treatment plan for certain types of cancers like prostate cancer.
2) **Adenocarcinoma**: Adenocarcinomas. Cancers that start in glandular tissues that make mucus or fluid, such as the lung, breast, prostate, or colon. Adenocarcinomas are considered a specific type (subtype) of carcinomas.
3) **Adenoma**: An adenoma is a benign (noncancerous) tumor. Adenomas start in the epithelial tissue, the tissue that covers your organs and glands. These tumors grow slowly and look like small mushrooms with a stalk
4) **Adjuvant therapy:** Treatment given after the main treatment to reduce the chance of cancer coming back by destroying any remaining cancer cells. It usually refers to chemotherapy, radiation therapy, hormone therapy, and/or immunotherapy given after surgery.
5) **Allogeneic stem cell transplant**
Uses bone marrow or stem cells from a donor whose tissue type closely matches that of the patient, to replace blood-forming cells that have been destroyed by disease or cancer treatment. This can be from a related donor or an unrelated donor.
6) **Benign:** Refers to a tumor that is not cancerous. The tumor does not usually invade nearby tissue or spread to other parts of the body.
7) **Biopsy:** This is the removal of a small section of the tumor, the sample will be analyzed by a histopathologist in order to

establish a precise diagnosis.

8) **Immunosuppressive** refers to treatments that turn down your body's <u>immune system</u> so it can't fight infections as well. People who are about to get a bone marrow or <u>organ transplant</u> get these therapies to keep their bodies from rejecting the new tissue.

9) **Immunotherapy** is treatment that stimulates the immune system to help the body fight diseases like cancer.

10) **In situ** describes cancer that hasn't spread to other tissue nearby.

11) **Malignant:** Cancerous, where the tumor grows uncontrollably and may spread.

12) **Localized**: A tumor restricted to a single site.

13) **Metastases**: Where the tumor has spread to other parts of the body beyond the primary site. Metastatic sites (secondaries) may be regional or distant from the original tumor.

14) **Neoadjuvant Therapy**: Neoadjuvant therapy is the administration of therapeutic agents (radiation therapy, chemotherapy) before the main treatment, such as surgery. The role of Neoadjuvant therapy is to allow for organ preservation in some case, to reduce the tumor size, making procedures (surgery) easier and increasing the likelihood of improved treatment outcomes.

15) **Staging:** This is a standardized system used to describe the extent and severity of the cancer. This provides critical information for treatment planning, prognosis estimation. The precise staging system used will depend on the type of cancer the patient has.

MYTHS SURROUNDING THE 'C' WORD

a)   Cancer is a Death Sentence

Despite the sobering statistics, Cancer is no longer a death sentence today. With better screening modalities, early detection, breakthroughs and continues advancements in cancer treatments, there is some reason to be optimistic even after getting the dreaded diagnosis. cancer is not always terminal. There are millions of people living with cancer today.

It is also worth noting that survival rates vary significantly depending on the stage and the type of cancer. When caught earlier, survival rates are encouraging: For instance, in the US The 5-year relative survival rate for stage 0 and 1 breast cancer is 99–100%. On the other hand, when metastatic, the statistics, though improving, are not so good; for example, the 5-year relative survival rate metastatic Liver and pancreatic cancers are less than 5%.

b)   All Cancers are the same and can be treated the same way

The makeup of each cancer is different and the was the cancer behaves in every individual is very different.

The way a pancreatic cancer cell will look and behave is different from the way a leukemia cancer cell with look and behave. Even more, different individuals, even with the same type of cancer, their cancer cells will look, behave and even have different genetic mutations.

Therefore a 'super cure' is unlikely and a 'one-size-fits-all' approach to cancer will not work. That is why even the best combination of treatments for each patient can produce very different results. A successful cancer treatment often involves a dedicated and experienced medical team to explore the options and map the most ideal path to recovery for that patient.

c) Cancer treatment hurts more than it cures

This may be due to the extreme side effects that people see in cancer patients undergoing chemotherapy and radiation therapy, but there is a belief that conventional cancer treatments are very harmful to the body and can sometimes cause more damage than the cancer itself. There are also those who believe that these treatments are useless in curing cancer and only end up creating severe discomfort before the cancer results in death.

One of the biggest reasons for this myth is because many cancers are found at a late stage and an aggressive course of treatment is usually needed to have a chance of recovery. At late stages of cancer, the disease would have spread to other places in the body and usually resulting in a very low survival rate. This, together with the severe side effects that aggressive chemotherapy and radiation therapy have, causes many people to doubt the effectiveness of conventional cancer treatments. The truth is that when cancer is diagnosed at an early stage, success rates using conventional treatment tend to be much higher. Those who are concerned about side effects should balance the importance of prolonging life with the quality of life when deciding about their treatment.

d) Surgeries and biopsies cause cancer to spread

During a biopsy, a small piece of tissue o sample of the suspected tumor is obtained so that a pathologist can examine it under a microscope and make a diagnosis. There are many different techniques for collecting a biopsy. For example, in a fine needle aspiration biopsy, the doctor inserts a needle attached to a syringe into the suspicious area to collect a small amount of tissue for diagnosis. In an excisional biopsy, the doctor removes the entire suspicious mass for examination. Surgery on the other hand, is usually done for Diagnosis, Staging, Tumor removal, Debulking, Palliation, Reconstructive surgery, or for preventive purposes.

Some people truly believe a biopsy could spread cancer through a process called 'Tumor seeding' or 'needle seeding'; which refers to rare occurrences when the needle inserted into a tumor during a biopsy dislodges and spreads cancer cells. Because the cancer cells grow along the needle's track, it has also been referred to as; needle track or tract seeding

The truth is, every medical procedure carries risks, and following a biopsy or surgery, some of these cancers could become more aggressive and recur. Studies have found that, this is because of the biology of cancer, not because of the biopsy or surgery. Many studies have also shown that tumor seeding only very rarely occurs, and that at the end of the day, the benefits of biopsies far outweigh the risks.

e) Superfoods Prevent Cancer

Superfoods have really become a term that is synonymous with ultra-healthy, nutrient-packed, plant-based foods and supplements. These are foods or beverages or ingredients that are essentially advertised as having exceptional powers, from fighting common health conditions to fighting cancer. Some foods like blueberries, beetroot, broccoli, garlic and green tea are known as cancer-preventing superfoods. These foods are certainly good for your health and are known to have positive effects in the fight against many diseases, e.g. containing antioxidants or helping to remove toxic elements in the body. However, it would be naive to look at any particular food as a protection against cancer. Everybody is different and cancer reacts differently in every person. There is no single food or food group that can provide enough protection against cancer. There is no denying the research showing that a healthy, balanced diet improves your health, and can even reduce your chance of developing cancer. However, there is no evidence that any specific diet or superfood cures cancer, despite many websites and videos that say otherwise.

f) It is better if you don't know you have cancer

I have had a lot of women finally come to the hospital months or even years after noticing a mass growing larger, and larger in their breast. To them, ignoring it will make the cancer 'less real'' and less powerful. That attitude did not change the fact that they had cancer and that the cancer was going to do what it does best; GROW'', whether they acted on it or not. Ignoring your cancer or signs of cancer will not make it go away. Instead, getting it worked up catching it early, may increase chances of catching it an early stage and treating or curing it. Cancer experts continue to emphasize the importance of routine cancer screenings, including mammograms, colonoscopies, and prostate exams.

g)   Only smokers get lung cancer

While it's true that tobacco use is the leading cause of lung cancer, and, Yes, most cases of lung cancer are linked to smoking tobacco, people who have never smoked can also be diagnosed with lung cancer. In fact, according to the American Cancer Society, about 20% of lung cancers deaths occur in people who have never smoked.

Your genetic make-up or family history can affect your risk of getting lung cancer. Exposure to substances such as asbestos, radon, uranium, arsenic and secondhand smoke can also increase the chance of developing lung cancer. There are also cases of lung cancer caused by scarring in the lung tissue due to previous illnesses and/or infections.

h)   If you don't have a family history of cancer, you are safe from cancer

Since cancer is largely caused by genetic defects in the DNA, many people believe that not having a family history of cancer means that they are very unlikely to develop cancer. In fact, only about 5 – 10% of cancer cases are caused by inherited genetic mutations. The remaining 90 – 95% of cases are caused by the individual's lifestyle and environment, like a smoking habit or exposure to cancer-causing chemicals. Still, people with a family history of cancer should get screened regularly and maintain a healthy lifestyle as they have a higher risk of developing cancer.

i)   Medical myth: natural cancer therapies can't harm you

This is one of the most misleading myths of modern medicine is that conventional cancer medications are not "natural" and so will be rejected by the body and that these artificial or "unnatural" cancer treatments are not good for you. These has created a lot of distrust between patient and their oncologist and has contributed to the popularity of unproven, alternative cancer treatments.

Today, many oncologists and other trained medical professionals are very open and supportive of any effective cancer treatments in any form, provided there is evidence to show they can work and are safe. An example is Laetrile; an extract from apricot kernels, which was, for years promoted as a natural alternative therapy for cancer; yet it is utterly useless for treating cancer and can cause fatal cyanide poisoning. Another example is the herb comfrey, which for many years, was recommended as an alternative cancer treatment; Modern scientific studies have found some evidence to support comfrey's use in treating minor wounds and joint pain, but oral preparations of the plant have also been linked to liver damage and cancer.

So, the notion of 'natural' does not necessarily equate to harmless. Nor does conventional necessarily equate to unnatural. Plenty of natural products are used in chemotherapy. Many studies suggest that alternative or complementary therapies, including some herbs, may help patients cope with the side effects of cancer treatment, no herbal products have been shown to be effective for treating cancer.

j)   You can 'catch' cancer

Cancer is not a contagious disease that spreads from person to person. In fact, you can hug, kiss and even be intimate with someone who has cancer and there will be no risk to you. The only situation that we know of so far, in which cancer can spread from one person to another is in the case of organ or tissue transplantation.; for example, a person who receives an organ or tissue from a donor who had cancer in the past may be at increased risk of developing a transplant-related cancer in the future. However, that risk is extremely low—about two cases of cancer per 10,000 organ transplants. Doctors avoid the use of organs or tissue from donors who have a history of cancer.

People who have had solid organ transplants (lung, heart, liver, kidney) have a small risk of developing cancer; usually as a result of the use of Immunosuppressive medicines; which on one hand, help prevent the immune system from rejecting the organ, but on the other hand, a weak immune system might fail to identify and eliminate abnormal cells.

In some people, cancers may be caused by certain viruses (some types of human papillomavirus, or HPV, for example) and bacteria (such as *Helicobacter pylori*). While a virus or bacterium can spread from person to person, the cancers they sometimes cause cannot spread from person to person.

There is already a cure for cancer out there; but the Drug companies are withholding these treatments from the general population for their own financial gains.

This is one of the most common myths out there and the one I get asked a lot. The key aspect I tell people to consider is this: if the issues also affects the ultra-rich people, then it is not a myth. Let's look at a few billionaires who died from cancer: Sheldon Adelson, Ali Broad, Randall Rollins, Wayne Hughes, Sheldon Solow, David Kock, and of course, Steve Jobs.

Scientific studies to determine the safety and effectiveness of new cancer treatments take time. I have seen many Doctors often go into cancer research because they have a family member or friend affected by the disease. They are as interested in finding a cure as anyone else, for the same reason — it affects them personally. They hate to see a loved one in pain and don't wish to lose this person. They also want to spare others what they have gone through.

SOMETHING TO REFLECT ON...

Sugar and Cancer: Nothing in excess can ever be good for the body, least of all sugar, which is known to cause diabetes and harm the bones. Sugar feeds all cells in the body, including cancer cells. Even when carbohydrates or sugar are not available, your body will make sugar from other sources, like protein or fat, to ensure your body and brain can function properly.

There is a connection between sugar and cancer risk, however, but it's more indirect than many realize. Eating a lot of high-sugar foods may mean more calories in your diet than you need, which eventually leads to excess body fat. So, the combined theory is that, excess sugar causes obesity which, in turn, leads to a pro-carcinogenic state (favorable for cancer development) in the body.

So, getting rid of sugar in the diet is not only challenging, but will not completely eliminate it from our body. The most important thing is to limit sugar to prevent weight gain which increases cancer risk. Focus on avoiding added sugars and choosing quality carbohydrates from whole food, plant-based sources.

The Future for Cancer and Cancer Care
During the past two to three decades, the model for cancer treatment has evolved from relatively non-specific cytotoxic agents to selective, targeted, mechanism-based therapeutics.

Cancer care has advanced at an impressive pace in recent years, and as we look down the road, the future of cancer and cancer care is not so grim. Immunotherapy will have been further developed, including personalized vaccines and combination of therapeutic vaccines with immune checkpoint inhibitors and targeted drugs.

In addition, adoptive T cell therapy and therapeutic vaccine combinations will have been developed and commercially established. I foresee precision medicine taking the lead. I foresee cancer becoming a chronic health condition like the way diabetes and hypertension are, today.

ABOUT THE AUTHOR

Ernestine is a seasoned expert in the field of oncology. Still practicing in the medical field as an oncology practitioner in one of the Nations' top cancer institutions, she currently has over 18 years of experience in cancer, research, cancer treatments, cancer diagnoses, cancer planning and cancer care. She holds a Doctorate of Nursing Practice degree, several oncology certifications and has dedicated her entire health professional career to advancing knowledge about cancer and how it affects patient and their families. Ernestine Muanya believes knowledge is power, and she is known for her raw passion for educating and empowering individuals to navigate the labyrinth of cancer with enthusiasm and confidence. Through this book, she hopes to share her knowledge to help demystify cancer and allow the facts be accessible to all.

64

List of References

American Cancer Society. Cancer Statistics Center. http://cancerstatisticscenter.cancer.org. Accessed November 10th, 2023.

American Cancer Society | Information and Resources about for Cancer: Breast, Colon, Lung, Prostate, Skin". www.cancer.org. Retrieved 11th November, 2023.

Acharya R, Mahapatra A, Verma HK, Bhaskar LVKS. Unveiling Therapeutic Targets for Esophageal Cancer: A Comprehensive Review. *Current Oncology*. 2023; 30(11):9542-9568. https://doi.org/10.3390/curroncol30110691

Clarke, M. A., Deshmukh, A. A., Suk, R., Roberts, J., Gilson, R., Jay, N., ... & Wentzensen, N. (2022). A systematic review and meta-analysis of cytology and HPV-related biomarkers for anal cancer screening among different risk groups. International Journal of Cancer, 151(11), 1889-1901.

Devico Marciano, N., Kroening, G., Dayyani, F., Zell, J. A., Lee, F. C., Cho, M., & Valerin, J. G. (2022). BRCA-mutated pancreatic cancer: from discovery to novel treatment paradigms. Cancers, 14(10), 2453.

Fedewa, S. A., Star, J., Bandi, P., Minihan, A., Han, X., Yabroff, K. R., & Jemal, A. (2022). Changes in cancer screening in the US during the COVID-19 pandemic. JAMA Network Open, 5(6), e2215490-e2215490.

Grapatsas K, Menghesha H, Dörr F, Baldes N, Schuler M, Stuschke M,

Darwiche K, Taube C, Bölükbas S. Pneumonectomy for Primary Lung Tumors and Pulmonary Metastases: A Comprehensive Study of Postoperative Morbidity, Early Mortality, and Preoperative Clinical Prognostic Factors. *Current Oncology*. 2023; 30(11):9458-9474. https://doi.org/10.3390/curroncol30110685

Islami, F., Guerra, C. E., Minihan, A., Yabroff, K. R., Fedewa, S. A., Sloan, K., ... & Jemal, A. (2022). American Cancer Society's report on the status of cancer disparities in the United States, 2021. CA: a cancer journal for clinicians, 72(2), 112-143.

Islam, M. R., Islam, F., Nafady, M. H., Akter, M., Mitra, S., Das, R., ... & Cavalu, S. (2022). Natural small molecules in breast cancer treatment: understandings from a therapeutic viewpoint. Molecules, 27(7), 2165.

Jourquin J, Reffey SB, Jernigan C, Levy M, Zinser G, Sabelko K, Pietenpol J, Sledge G Jr. Susan G. Komen Big Data for Breast Cancer Initiative: How Patient Advocacy Organizations Can Facilitate Using Big Data to Improve Patient Outcomes. JCO Precis Oncol. 2019 December 11th, 2023. doi: 10.1200/PO.19.00184. PMID: 32923852; PMCID: PMC7446366.

Li S, Miller-Wilson LA, Guo H, Fisher DA. Adherence to colorectal cancer screening and healthcare resource utilization: a longitudinal analysis in Medicare beneficiaries aged 66-75 years. Curr Med Res Opin. 2022;38(12):2201-2208. doi: 10.1080/03007995.2022.2133493.

Patel S, Brennan K, Zhang L, Djerboua M, Nanji S, Merchant S, Flemming J. Colorectal Cancer in Individuals with Cirrhosis: A Population-Based Study Assessing Practice Patterns, Outcomes, and Predictors of Survival. *Current Oncology*. 2023; 30(11):9530-9541. https://doi.org/10.3390/curroncol30110690

Sathiyapalan A, Baloush Z, Ellis PM. Update on the Management of Stage III NSCLC: Navigating a Complex and Heterogeneous Stage of Disease. *Current Oncology*. 2023; 30(11):9514-9529. https://doi.org/10.3390/curroncol30110689

Shah R, Polen-De C, McGree M, Fought A, Kumar A. Re-Evaluating Chemotherapy Dosing Strategies for Ovarian Cancer: Impact of Sarcopenia. *Current Oncology*. 2023; 30(11):9501-9513.

https://doi.org/10.3390/curroncol30110688

The NCCN Biomarkers Compendium® © 2022 National Comprehensive Cancer Network, Inc. Available at: NCCN.org. Accessed [December 17th, 2023].

Thomas PB, Alinezhad S, Joshi A, Sweeney K, Tse BWC, Tevz G, McPherson S, Nelson CC, Williams ED, Vela I. Introduction of Androgen Receptor Targeting shRNA Inhibits Tumor Growth in Patient-Derived Prostate Cancer Xenografts. *Current Oncology*. 2023; 30(11):9437-9447. https://doi.org/10.3390/curroncol30110683

Yaffe MJ, Mainprize JG. Effect of Breast Screening Regimen on Breast Cancer Outcomes: A Modeling Study. *Current Oncology*. 2023; 30(11):9475-9483. https://doi.org/10.3390/curroncol30110686

www.ingramcontent.com/pod-product-compliance
Lightning Source LLC
Chambersburg PA
CBHW050849260726
48660CB00006B/2531